I am a Vegetarian

By Olayinka Ladeji

Acknowledgements

All Glory is due to Neter (God) for the inspiration for this book.
Love and thanks to my families—spiritual, blood, and otherwise.
Special thanks to Senbeb Café of Washington, D.C, USA

This book is dedicated to my Beloved daughter, S-Utchai Maa-t, my other beloved babies, and children the world over who give me every reason to put "pen to paper". May you be brought up to live as God's likeness.

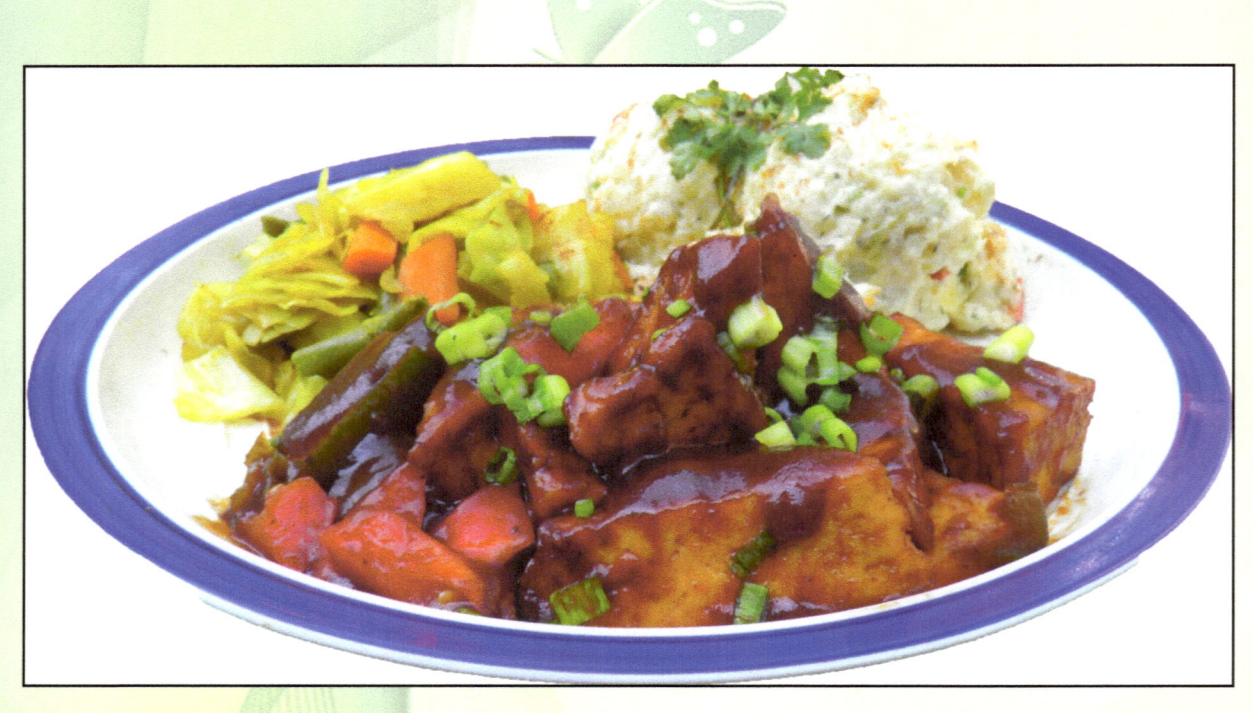

I am a vegetarian. Yes I am.

I eat a natural diet. Yes I do.

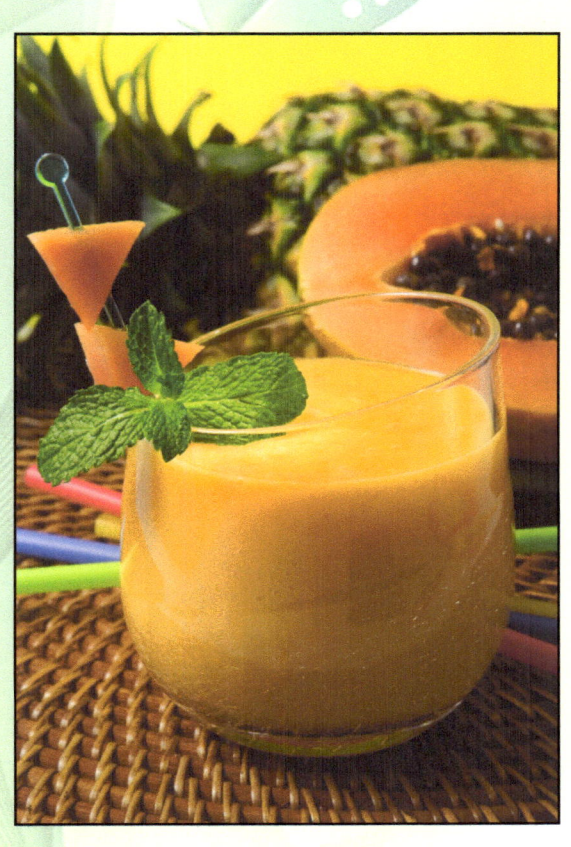

In the morning I drink a protein shake,

Yum, yum, yum...now I'm wide awake.

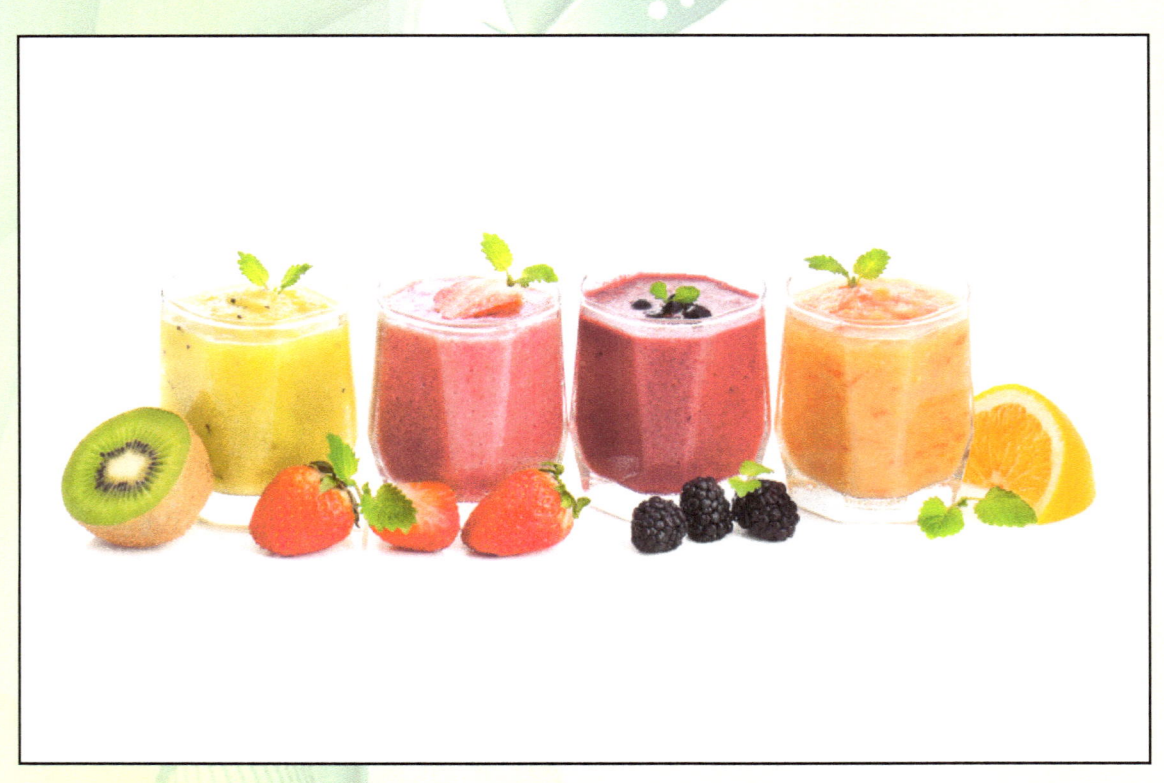

It has nut milk, protein powder, lecithin,
flax, nut butter, a banana without the skin.

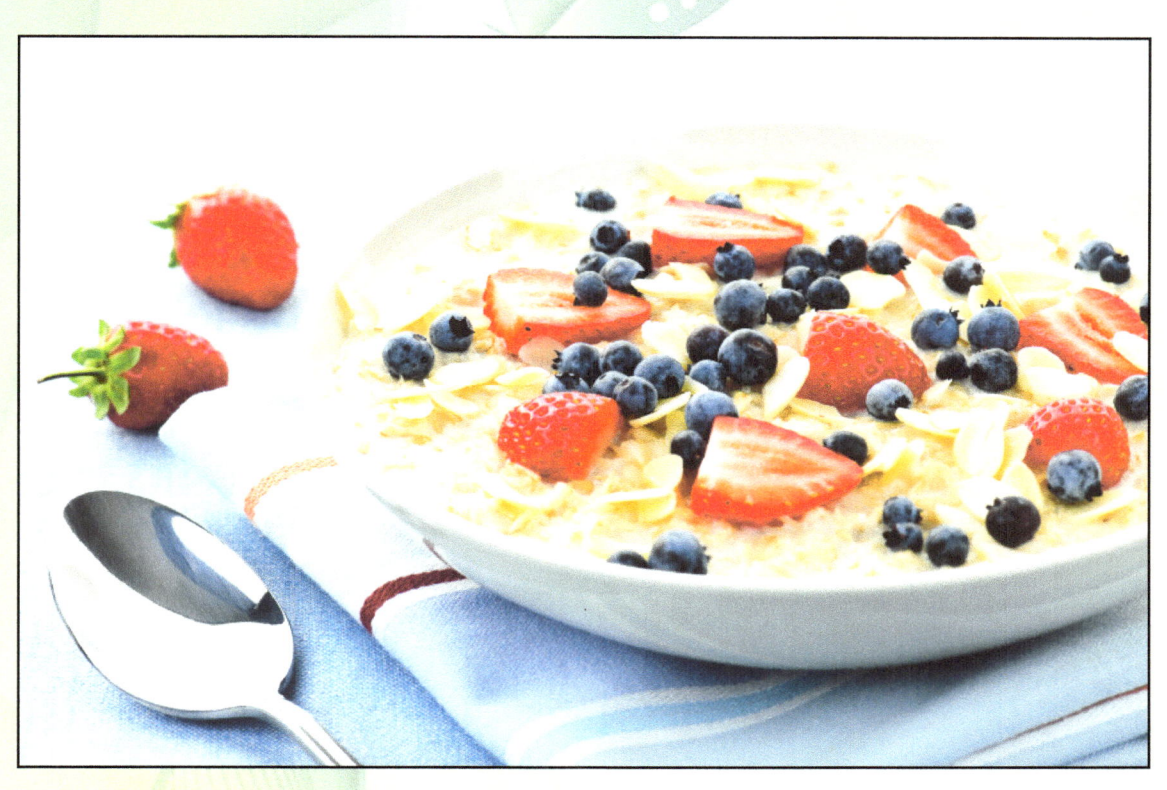

And I munch, munch, munch

on my bowl of oat groats.

I say "Tua Neter" (Thank God), this has my vote.

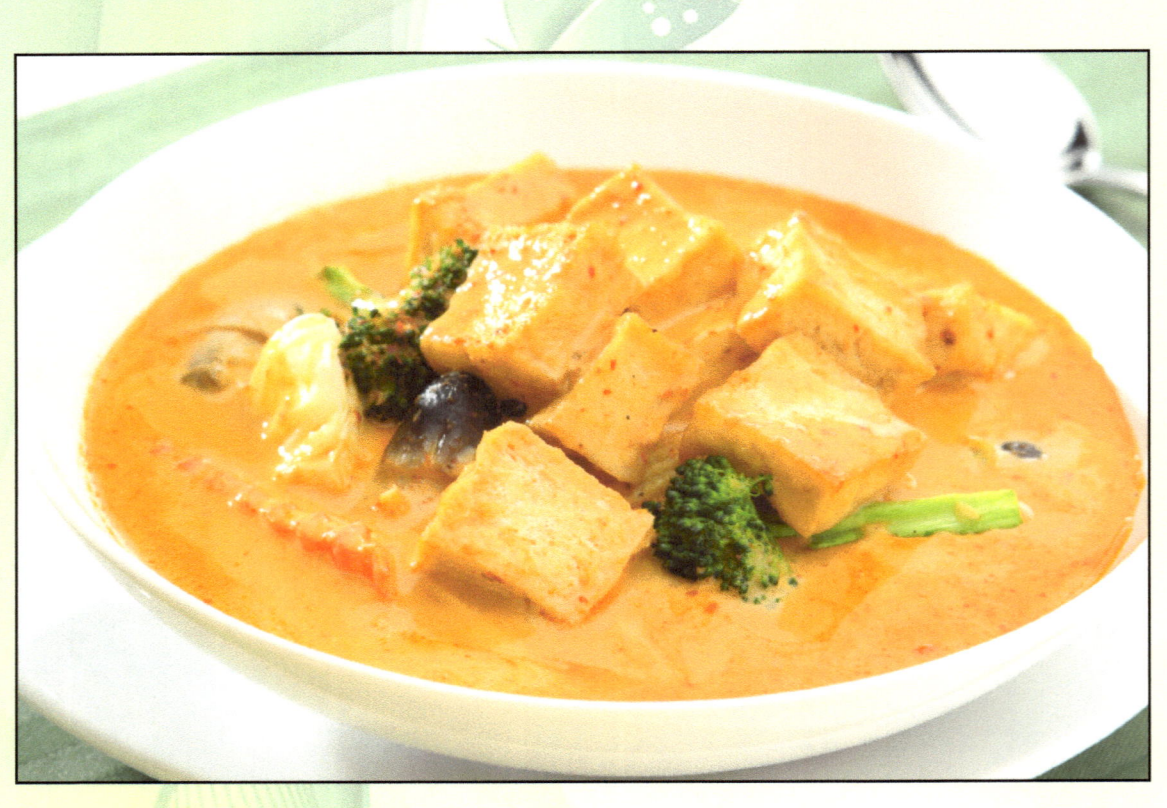

I eat raw nuts, lentils and some beans –
Even tofu or moi-moi for protein.

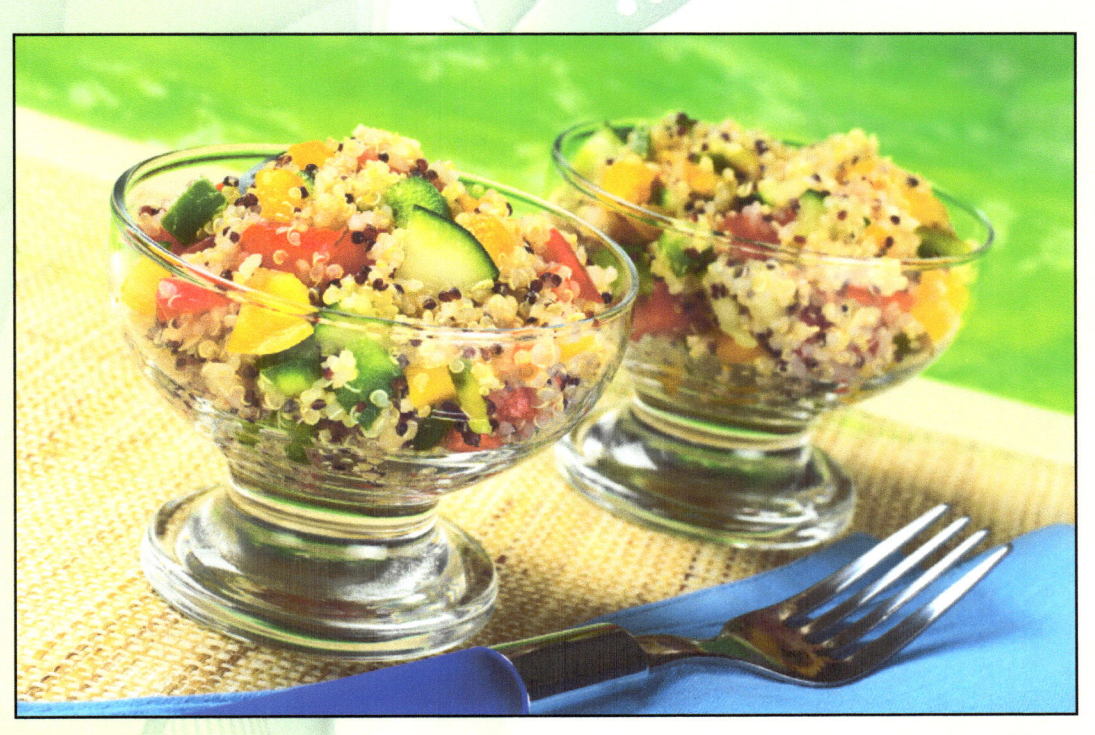

I eat brown rice, barley, and quinoa for grains.

My food is yummy and none remains.

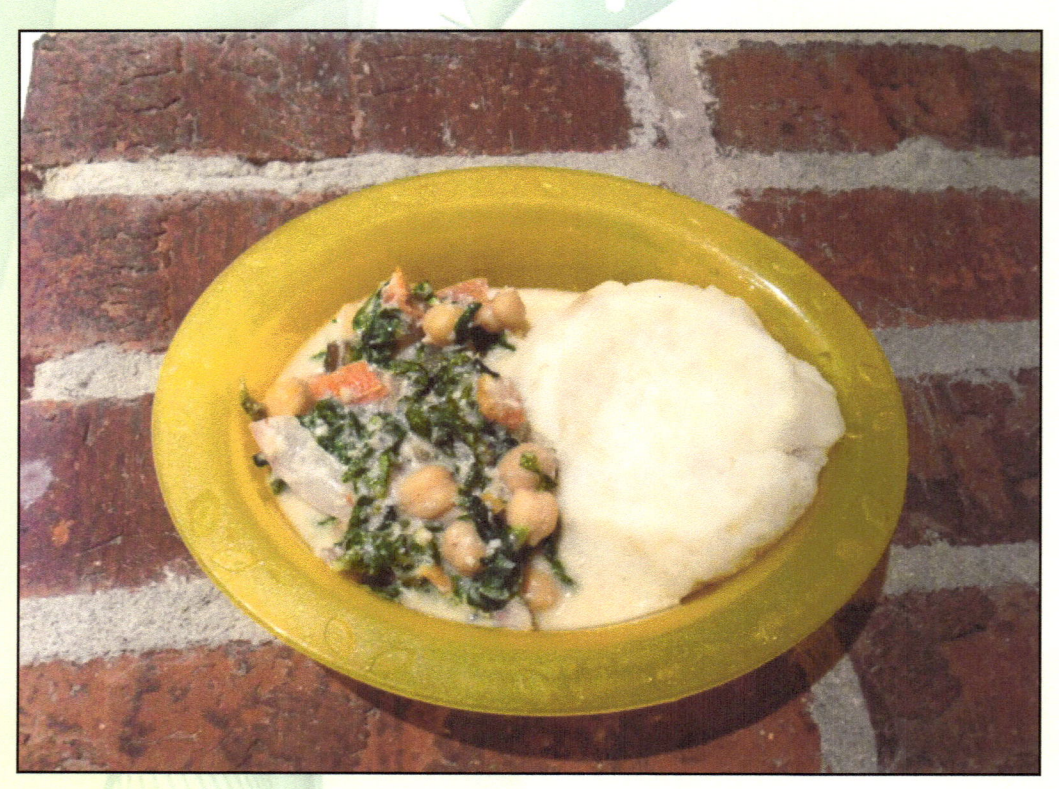

Some days I have some pounded yam
or plantain or cassava, Blessed I am!

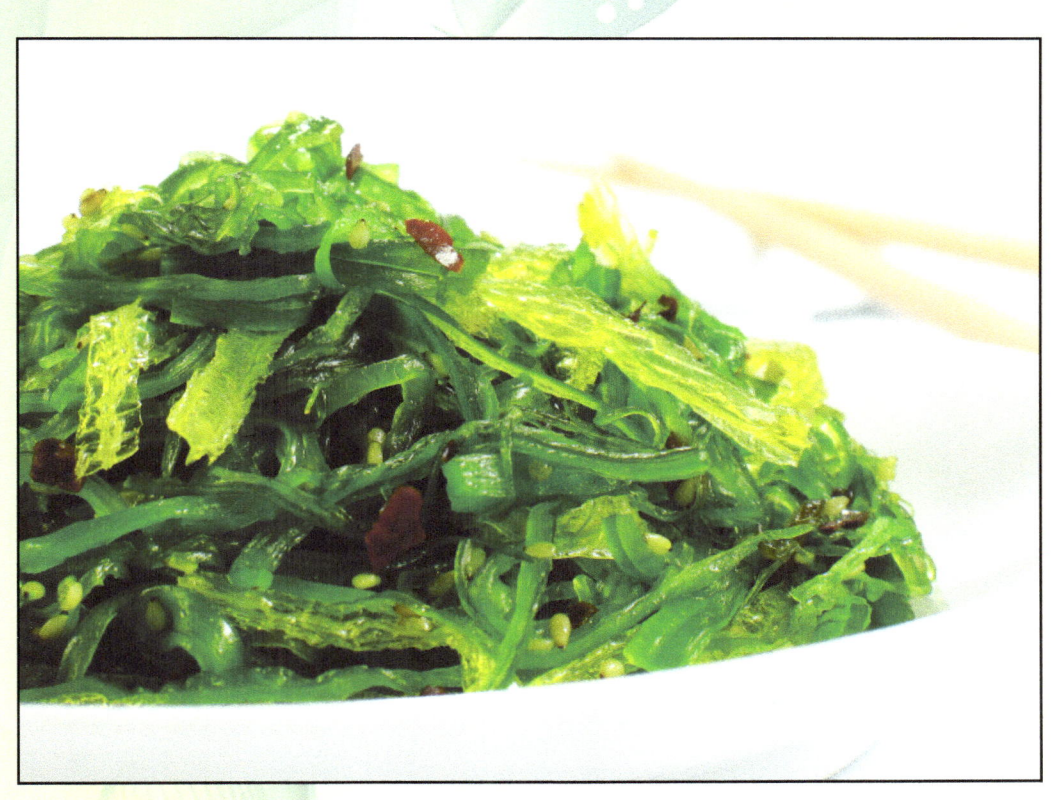

I eat different types of salads and vegetables.

Callaloo, kale and spinach make me so full.

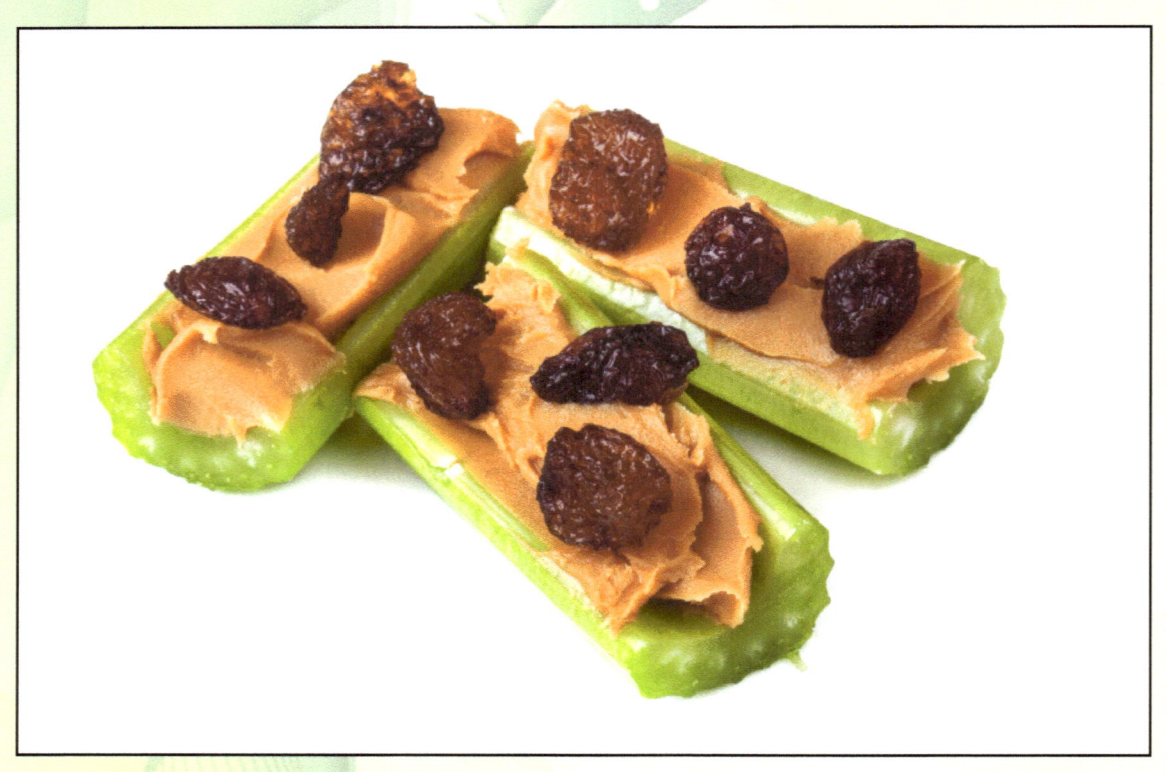

Broccoli and squash are my favorite picks.

I gobble down collard greens and celery sticks.

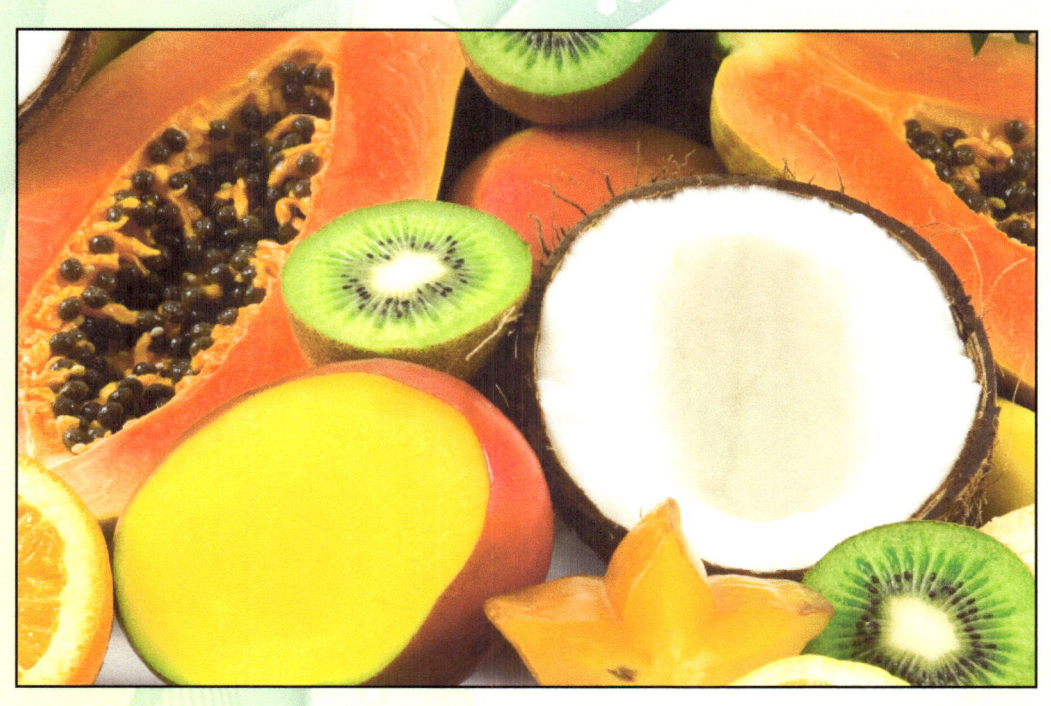

For snacks I eat lots of fresh organic fruit.

Vitamins and supplements, in my mouth I put.

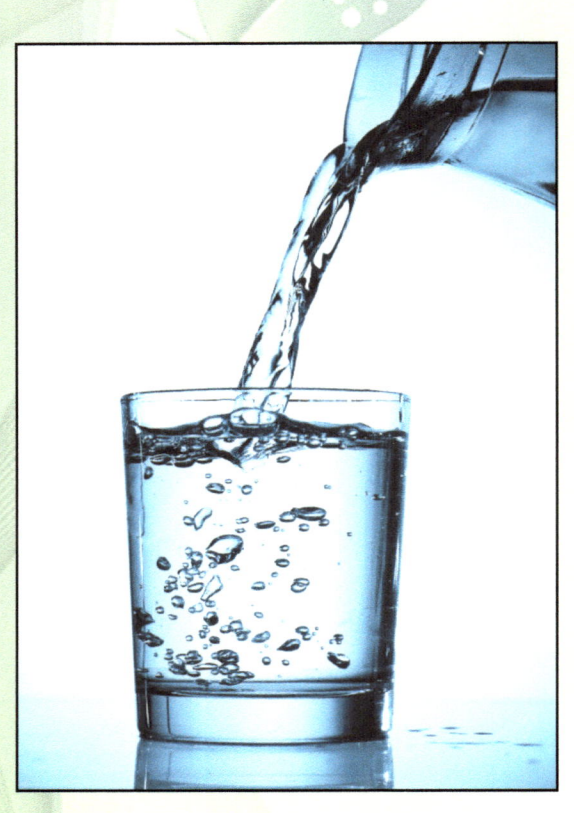

And I sip, sip, sip on water and juice

throughout the day.

Gets me in the mood to play, play, play.

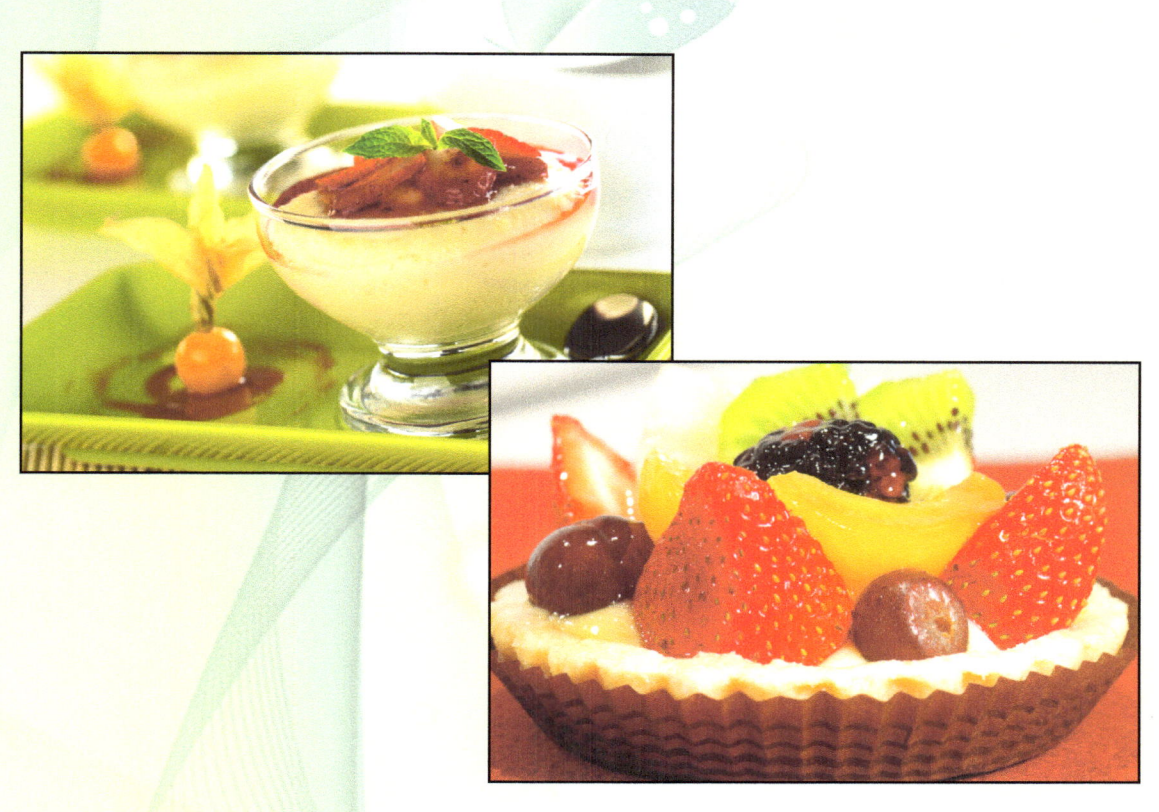

I love my organic diet. I love what I eat.

It makes my body healthy and strong, doesn't it?

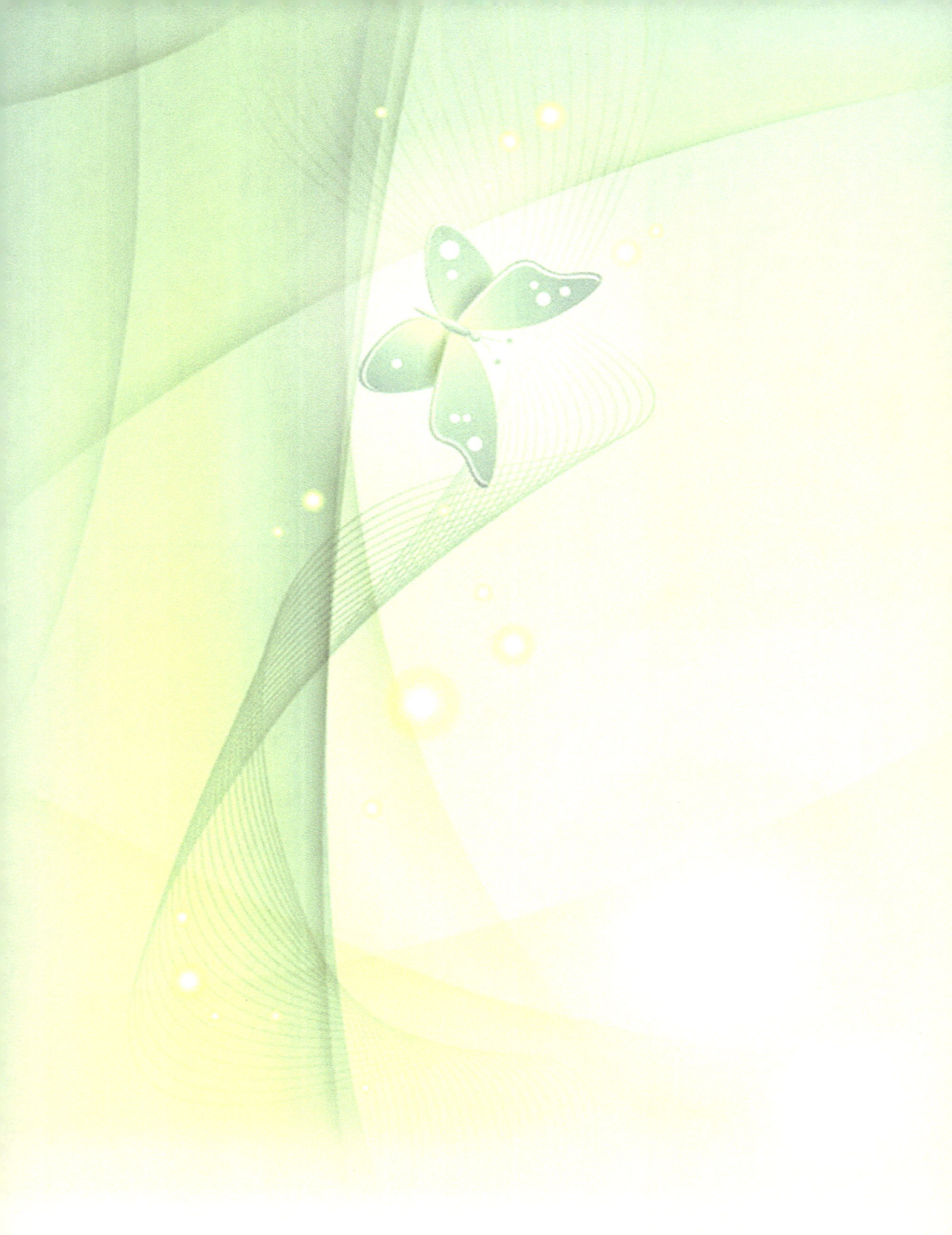

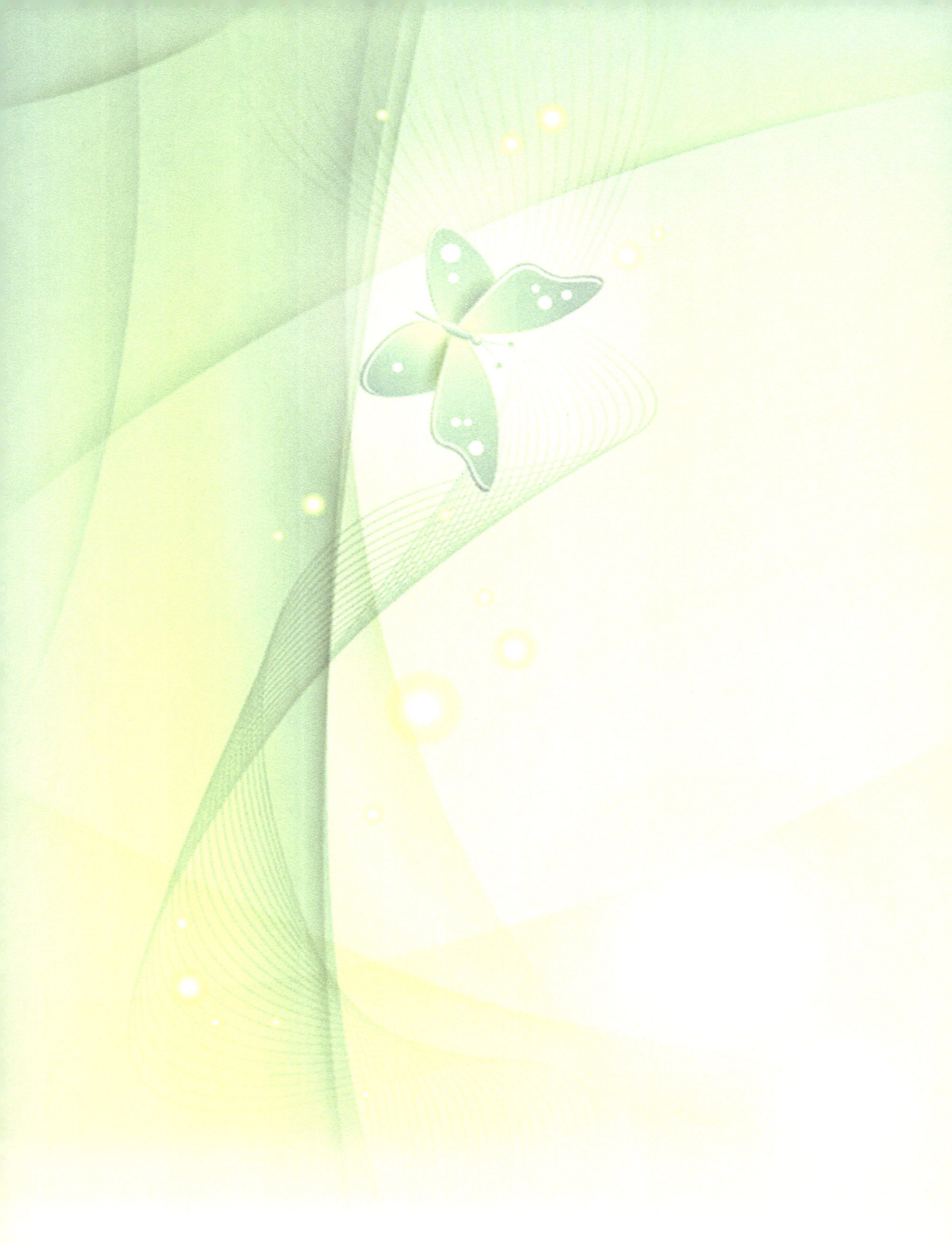

www.ingramcontent.com/pod-product-compliance
Lightning Source LLC
Chambersburg PA
CBHW060824290526
45792CB00005BB/1788